THE BODY BEAUTIFUL

YOUR ULTIMATE FITNESS AND WEIGHT LOSS GUIDE

BY BARRY LUDLOW

I0429149

COPYRIGHT

The Body Beautiful

ACKNOWLEDGEMENT

This book and all it contains has evolved from years of education, knowledge and experience. Everything the author has achieved over the years has only been made possible through unconditional love, support and advice from the authors mother Mrs Ellie Ludlow and father Mr Patrick Ludlow. The author would like them to realise just how much they mean to him, how much he appreciates their support and therefore has decided to dedicate this book to them.

FOREWORD-BARRY LUDLOW. BSc HONS, PGCE, M.ED.

The author is a passionate sports-man who has combined his love of sports with education having gained a Bachelor of Science honours Degree in Sport, exercise sciences and leisure, a PGCE in Physical education and a Masters Degree in Education. In addition to this the author has been a teacher of physical education, science and sports science for nine years as well as coaching individuals and teams for fifteen years. This experience blended with education and sporting knowledge has given the author a real insight in to all aspects of training as well as how to achieve the best results. The author's credibility is proven through academic and personal achievements and through the results this book will deliver for you.

TABLE OF CONTENTS

Chapter One-Smarter training

Chapter Two-The FITT Principal

Chapter Three-Programs

Chapter Four-Nutrition

Chapter Five-Components of Fitness

Chapter Six- Lifestyle

WARNING

Not all exercise programs are suitable for everyone so please consult your Doctor before beginning any exercise program. You should always warm-up for a few minutes before any workout and you should never exercise beyond the level you feel comfortable with. Some of the exercises, which are included are quite difficult and should not be attempted by someone who does not meet minimum fitness levels or by someone who has not exercised for a long time. Anyone with a history of knee, hip, shoulder, back or neck problems should also get permission from their Doctor before beginning any of the exercise programs included. This warning is not to be discounted as there are many fitness alternatives if you have weaknesses or are prone to injuries. The reader and possible user therefore assume all risk of injury or harm of any kind in the use of any of the programs or sessions included in this book. If at any time you feel you are exercising beyond your current fitness levels or feel discomfort of any kind such as dizziness or nausea then you should discontinue exercising immediately and reconsider the use of any exercise routine included in this book.

CHAPTER ONE
SMARTER TRAINING

Are you content with your body? I think it is fair to assume since you are reading this book that you need some help as do most people and the good news for you is this book can help you achieve a body you have only dreamt about. Have you often looked at others wishing you had a body like theirs? Most people are guilty of this and off course some people have an advantage in terms of genes, wealth and spare time however it is possible to control your body shape and gain results you never thought were possible. This book will give you the tools to make these results possible. Many people suffer from weight and body issues, this book will tackle these issues in terms of arming readers with clear methods helping them achieve goals and results they have only dreamed off. The following chapters will look at a variety of ways to lose weight as well as your overall health and well being. Obviously your choice of method will depend on what you want to achieve but one thing will be constant and that is the enormous sense of well being from physical and mental confidence you will receive while living inside your new body. Let's get started on the road to you becoming body beautiful.

Specific

When choosing a training regime you will need to have a goal or target in mind, which will enable you to use appropriate and specific methods in order to achieve the outcome you desire. This may seem confusing so I will use an example to ensure you realise it is basic common sense that you and others can apply to your training regime. A top class tennis player's goal will be to win major tournaments, which requires him to be in peak physical condition meaning he will need the main elements of fitness including power, muscular endurance, endurance, strength, flexibility and agility. Although these are all important it would be foolish for him to pack on too much muscle in order to increase his strength as he needs to remain lean and not be carrying excess weight which would affect the other elements. Therefore it is important to be specific in the training so as to find the correct balance overall. His program would be designed to meet his overall goal and still be very much tailored around tennis and the sports requirements such as speed around the court, changing direction quickly, power, flexibility and the dexterity involved in the shot making. Another example would be a marathon runner who should not bulk up too much in terms of muscle as they cannot afford to carry excess weight and should not incorporate too much anaerobic training into their regime as their sport is endurance based. Your program should be tailored around your sporting needs and individual goals. Think about what you really want to achieve and get out of your sporting performance and then you will have a better idea of how to go about fulfilling those ambitions and what road to choose to get you there. Specific training methods can be used to improve each of the fitness elements. Some examples of these methods include:

Continuous-Sustained periods of regular training without rest. This cardiovascular based fitness training includes swimming, cycling and running.

Circuits-This training involves moving from station to station at various paces for various times in a special order known as a circuit.

Cross training-This is when an athlete uses another sport and its training methods and applies this in their own sport. Skills and fitness elements are transferred.

Weight training-Improving strength and endurance in the muscles using resistance and the appropriate number of repetitions and sets.

Fartlek-This type of training involves lots of running, walking skiing or cycling at varying speeds enhancing both anaerobic and aerobic capacity.

Interval-Training involving high intensity bursts of exercise alternated with low intensity or rest. Muscular endurance and speed are improved. This type of training is also very good for fat loss without losing too much muscle if done correctly.

Altitude-This requires training above sea level, where there is less oxygen available. When training aerobically in this way fitness will improve very quickly along with aerobic capacity.

In order to train efficiently and specifically you must work out your current level of fitness, amount of aerobic or anaerobic training your sport requires and be able to calculate target zones and thresholds of training. For example you can use maximum heart rate (MHR) to calculate exactly how hard you and your heart need to work in order to improve both aerobic and anaerobic fitness. Your MHR is calculated by subtracting your age from 220. Aerobic fitness is improved by working at 60-80% of MHR.

Aerobic. Only by working inside your aerobic target zone at 60-80% as mentioned above can you improve your overall aerobic fitness. When you reach a minimum of 60% you cross what is known as your aerobic threshold the heart rate above which you gain aerobic fitness.

Anaerobic can be improved by working inside your anaerobic target zone, which is between 80-100% of your MHR. Benefits include increased strength, power and muscular-endurance. Anaerobic threshold is crossed when you reach a minimum of 80% of your MHR. Working anaerobically you create what is known as an oxygen debt and can only keep going for a short period of time. Oxygen debt is the amount of oxygen taken in during recovery above that which would normally be taken in during rest. This is a result of a shortage of available oxygen during exercise. Post exercise it is always a good idea to record your heart rate so you can assess your fitness levels as this gives you a good indication of your recovery rate. The faster your heart rate returns to normal the fitter you are. MHR will depend on your levels of training, age and other contributing factors so are very individually based.

Measurable

Once you have established your overall goal and are happy with it you must stay focused. This is why you must make your goals measurable as having measurable goals means ensuring that you can monitor progress at various times. After all who will achieve success or can monitor an unclear vision or goal when you do not know what to look for, what to change or even if you are on the right road. You will undoubtedly become disillusioned and fail if your goal is not crystal clear in your mind. If your goal is to lose weight then set a number such as 20 pounds in four months and check your weight at regular intervals. It is important to point out that muscle weight and water retention plays a part in overall body weight and it is possible to lose inches off the waist without the scales reflecting this to a large extent. Therefore you can be achieving results, which are just as important as your original goal and it is important not to become weight obsessed. There is no exact weight to be body beautiful.

Having measurable goals is an extension of having specific goals. Through measuring your training effectively, you will be able to see tangible results and progress towards achieving your overall goal. The author recommends checking and measuring your progress every six weeks.

Attainable

It's good to set specific goals and monitor your progress however if your goals are not reachable then you will fail. Setting appropriate realistic targets will ensure you build confidence as you go as you will feel good about achieving each target and these steps will lead to overall success. It is important to point out that when setting these targets that although they have to be realistic they must not be too easy as this will not feel like an achievement and have very little benefits. For example if you are twelve stone eleven pounds and you set a goal of reaching twelve stone seven pounds this is not a real challenge to you and will have limited benefits. Instead it would be better to aim for the twelve stone zero pounds mark, which would have increased benefits and be a real achievement. It is about finding the correct balance for you personally. An attainable goal should challenge you, make you commit to it, and the goal should produce a feeling of success when it's achieved.

Get Real!

Being realistic as much as it pains people is important as it is simply not possible to achieve some dreams and every individual has their own skill set and genetics. However just because some of you will never make the Olympics, champions league, Wimbledon or the rugby world cup final except maybe to watch it does not mean that some other dreams you have cannot be achieved. Setting targets or goals based on dreams can be difficult. Therefore you should ask yourself the following questions; Have I got the skill set to achieve my goal, do I have any illnesses or limitations, which will affect my training, do I believe as objectively as possible that I can achieve this goal/target, do I really want to achieve this goal and how will I feel when I do, am I setting the goals for myself or are they based on the opinions of others? This is especially important as you should not place too much importance into opinions and advice from friends as sometimes they do not always have your best interests at heart and even if they do their knowledge and understanding of training and body issues is somewhat lacking. Think about what you and only you want to achieve and only use the advice of experts such as the author or another reputable personal trainer for guidance. This will ensure that your goals are realistic, measurable, specific and most of all achievable. You will then be completely happy with the results you achieve.

Time

What most people do not realise is that the time you put into exercising and the numbers of times you train in every week are very important. Consistent training and incorporating it into your routine are vital in order to achieve the best results and that body you have always wanted. The reason most people do not achieve the results they were aiming for is usually down to a lack of commitment over a sustained period of time. You will all have seen an influx of people in your local gym after Christmas armed with their new year's resolutions and training with quite a lot of effort to begin with only for the novelty to fade along with their desire to achieve their goals. This is because they realise that there is hard work required and a pre requisite to commit for the long term. Therefore do not make the same mistake of obsessing over an idea or particular workout, training hard for a few weeks only to give up after a short period of time. Instead chose a training method or methods which suits you and you know you can work into your lifestyle and routine. You do not have to commit a lot of time if the training is done correctly as it is about quality not quantity as the old saying goes and this is where this book will keep you on the right track giving you a guideline of how long and how often you should train as well as the intensity. How long you train for is very important as if training is too short without the intensity it will not work, too long and you will burn out and find it difficult to sustain for periods of time. Training for an optimal time you will feel energised after a workout although it will be tough during and you will achieve optimal results. I must reiterate again here how important consistency is as even if you are training for the correct amount of time you cannot expect to gain results if you do not train over a consistent number of days every week. We can all easily find excuses not to train on certain days and some days will have to be missed, which is understandable but what is not acceptable is making excuses on a regular basis because those who have the body beautiful and achieve the best results stick and commit to their training on a regular basis with no excuses for the most part. I have often heard people say things like I just do not have the time to train or they do not have all the responsibilities I have, I don't know where they get the time, lucky them, I wish I had so much time on my hands, they obviously do not have as many things to do with their day as I have, sound familiar? Most of the high level trainers that I know and have trained with will make time in their day to train and they all have very busy high profile jobs where their time is precious. Most of them have families too which makes it difficult but they still find enough time to maintain the physique which they worked so hard to achieve. There should be no excuse for the most part as everyone can find even 5-12 minutes in their day which is all you need for some forms of training, which can also be done at home. I will give you some of these exercises later in the book. Once you have experienced the results exercise brings you such as better health, fitness, tone and definition, self confidence, mental discipline and stress relief you will definitely make time for exercise as you will not want to go back to living any other way. None of us like deadlines but when you set a time limit to a goal or target you have something to aim for and an inner pressure to get things done especially towards the closing stages. This extra motivation is good as you know you are so close to your dream. You will need to stick with your original deadline and you must take stock of your results on that day through means of a relevant fitness test. Even if you have fallen short for some reason you therefore have experience and a guideline of the timeframe involved in achieving your goal and what you need to do differently in the future thanks to your fitness tests every six weeks along the way. Your time and commitment is an investment but one well worth making.

Putting it all Together

Using SMART principles is a well-known guideline in the world of physical education, in your goal setting and training plan does not have to be difficult or cut into your workout time. The reasoning behind using smart principles is to give you a clear understanding and road to follow. You will not be turning up at the gym and thinking what I should do today; instead you will have a plan with specific training days giving you clarity and keeping you focused on your goals to drive you forward. It is important to review how you are getting on throughout your training. My advice is to monitor your progress every six weeks to ensure your body is shocked into continuously producing results and not plateauing. This can be done through fitness tests or simply by looking at recordings of your progress from the start. For example weight lifted, repetitions made, body fat lost and difference in appearance. Small changes should be made in order to achieve this every six weeks. Obviously if there is anything wrong with your training and this becomes apparent during the six weeks you should make the relevant changes and adapt accordingly. Six weeks is a good balance in terms of allowing a long enough time frame for noticeable results without things becoming stale? It is the correct time to make adjustments, which we will look at in greater detail later in the book. Do not fret too much if you fall a little short the first time. Experience with goal-based training plans will help you better understand how much time it takes to accomplish a specific task. Finally, have some fun. This shouldn't turn you into a robot. All you've done is set a clear goal and planned out how you're going to reach it. Quick fix training plans rarely if ever contribute to long-term success. Achieving goals is not a quick process. Do not fret if you are not achieving your goals as fast as you would like because if you follow the plan and commit to it making the relevant changes at the correct stages you can only succeed. Also what most people do not realise is that everybody hits a plateau when training or trying to lose weight and this is due to the following. When you begin a training program there is usually an initial burst of weight loss as your body is not used to the training and responds by using its glycogen stores in the muscles, which holds on to water and therefore most of the weight shed at the start is water. After a few weeks your body's metabolism slows down so it is important to increase your level of activity and cut down bad calorie intake. This is why it is so important to use the SMART principles to make changes and review your training program every six weeks in order to achieve the best possible results. So you are all clear SMART has a number of slightly different variations which can be used in conjunction with your goal setting.

S=Specific, significant, stretching

M=Measurable, meaningful, motivational

A=Attainable

R=Realistic

T=Time-based, timely, tangible, trackable

The SMART principle if applied correctly will help you achieve your goal which will also improve your life. Throughout the process of achieving your body beautiful you will be improving your self confidence self discipline and physical appearance as well as your overall health and well-being.

CHAPTER TWO
FITT PRINCIPLE

F=Frequency

In the wake of any form of fitness training, the body goes through a process of rebuilding muscle and restoring energy reserves used during exercise. The frequency of training involves establishing the correct balance so that the body is worked out effectively and at the same time giving you enough time to recover before your next session. One factor many people do not take into consideration is the demands they are under on a day to day basis outside of training. For example you're working hours and intensity, looking after children and various other commitments. Therefore your training should be chosen so you can tailor your workouts around your other commitments at a level which will not push you too far. Age and health also have to be taken into consideration and there will be tips on this throughout this book but any personal trainer who knows what he or she is doing should have already factored all this into account before giving you a programme.

Aerobic conditioning.

The author recommends between three and six sessions per week preferably five as this will give you the consistency of training required to achieve the elusive body beautiful results which include superb definition, low body fat, heart and lung benefits, increased efficiency, weight loss and maintenance for a great look. Elite athletes who train more than this still need to leave enough recovery time and they have advantages over others including being professional therefore having more time, their high fitness, talent levels and one to one expert coaching therefore it is not a good idea for anyone else to train in this way more than five or six times a week as it could be very detrimental to their health.

Resistance Training

This type of training, which involves resistance such as weights or bodyweight exercises requires the correct amount of rest between sessions, which is just as important as the training itself. An example of this would be a total body workout in the gym using free weights, which works all the muscles, this should be performed three times weekly allowing at least 48 hours recovery between sessions so muscles can fully repair themselves thus achieving maximum results. Resistance training must be tailored around the individual and their goals. For example someone wishing to work one or two muscle groups each day they are in the gym could train as often as six days per week as the muscles worked the previous day are getting to rest and are not the focus on that particular day. Although it is important to point out that despite only working perhaps two body parts you are still exerting your body in general, I.e. Major organs. Also someone wishing to add or maintain muscle while shedding body fat may consider using circuit style weight training where they move from station to station without much rest thus keeping the heart rate and metabolic rate high helping them to shed fat. It is important to design the correct number of relevant stations and the time between stations for the individual. This along with the best forms of resistance training will be documented later in the book.

I=Intensity

The I in the FITT principle refers to intensity. This is the amount of effort which needs to be invested in a session and the programme in general. You must not try too much as you will burn out but equally you must exert enough effort so as your body will adapt and make the necessary changes. Again this is about finding the correct balance for you and is dependent on the type of training you will select. In order to measure or monitor your training intensity your heart rate can be a great guideline. Through having a pulse rate monitor with you or on you it can relay your current heart rate to you constantly so the training can be adapted accordingly. These are also useful for monitoring your heart rate before and after training to establish how quickly you recover. Heart rate monitoring is used regularly to measure intensity in aerobic endurance training to ensure the person in question is working in their target zone. This zone is established through your fitness level and age but can be quickly worked out using the following method.

Heart Rate & Maximum Heart Rate

Once you know how to take your heart rate by measuring beats per minute and using your neck or wrist to do so then you can calculate your target zone by subtracting your age from 220 which is now your maximum heart rate. If you are 20 this means your maximum heart rate is 200 and if you are just beginning to exercise you have to work out what 50-70% of 200 is, which in this case is between 100-140 beats per minute and work at an intensity between the two for good results. If you are already involved in playing sport or an athlete your target heart rate should be at the heart rate zone of between 70-85% of your maximum. This is between 140-170 beats per minute in the case of a twenty year old.

T=Type

The first T in FITT refers to the type of exercise or training you choose to do in order to gain the results you want.

The first example is Cardio respiratory training as this type of training improves your cardiovascular system and uses the main muscle groups. Swimming, running, cycling, walking are all good examples.

The second example I will use is resistance training. When people hear or see the word resistance they automatically think of weights which are a great form of exercise with many benefits but there are other forms of resistance training. For example circuits, bodyweight exercises such as press ups, sit ups and also the use of resistance bands which are good for recreating sporting situations and techniques, which you can then practice from the comfort of your own home.

There are other types of training which will again be examined in greater detail later in the book. For now it is more important that you understand the principles involved with training.

T=Time

The second T in FITT refers to time and how long each of your sessions is as well as the overall time involved in your programme before making changes. For example in resistance training you should not train for any more than 45-60 minutes. In the author's opinion and experience any more than 45 minutes has very limited benefits and any training over 60 minutes has been proved many times to have detrimental effects on the body as well as increasing your risk of injury. It is also important to note that the initial hour post exercise is a crucial time to take on board some carbohydrates and protein as this can aid recovery time and reduce muscle soreness. Also equally important is the rest time you give yourself between resistance sessions, which should be 48 hours for best results. In terms of Cardio training people who are not particularly fit should begin by exercising in their target heart rate zone for between 20-30 minutes and no more until their fitness levels increase in which case they can exercise for up 45-60 minutes. Again unless you are an elite level athlete or a marathon runner any more than 60 minutes is usually of little benefit. The overall timeframe involved should work in six week blocks where you look at making the necessary changes to your programme in order to achieve the best results. It can take up to a year to achieve peak performance but by examining results and your programme every six weeks you can keep on top of your training and your goals and stimulate your body into making the changes you want.

The FITT principle applies to most people however Sports specific athletes will normally use another set of principles. These are as follows; Specificity, Overload, Adaption, Progression, Reversibility and Variation.

Specificity

Specificity basically refers to the specific mobility requirements of a particular sport. A coach may for example analyse the techniques involved in an athlete's sport or event determining which joint actions are involved and how that athlete's range of movement can be improved. For instance a thrower may need increased mobility in his or her shoulder and spine. Basically if you can remember to incorporate relevant training techniques which focus on areas of joint mobility which your sport uses then you are on the right path. A top tennis player is not going to be concentrating a lot of time to his hip mobility if it is already good he will instead look to strengthen perhaps his shoulder joint mobility which is also relevant but needs extra work. He will also be looking to increase his strength in ways which will help his tennis by using various techniques such as replicating tennis movements using forms of resistance. Specificity refers to training relevant muscle groups and fitness elements suited to your sport or training goals. For example; A sprinter is not going to be concentrating on endurance work to improve when his or her sport is anaerobic based.

Overload

A muscle will only strengthen when forced to operate beyond its normal intensity. Overloading of the muscles must be progressively increased at the correct times usually every six weeks in order to stimulate adaptive responses that you want. Overload can be progressed through the following methods, increasing resistance, usually in small increments so as to avoid injury, increasing the number of repetitions, increasing the number of sets of the exercise and increasing the intensity, which is basically more work or effort in the same allocated time frame or you can reduce recovery times.

Recovery

Rest is as important for achieving results and adaption of the muscles as the training is. Your body needs time to recover and repair the muscles used during exercise.

Adaption

Adaption takes place during the recovery period when the training session is finished. This is where the body reacts to the stress and training loads it has been placed under and adapts accordingly enabling you to perform at these higher levels long term. This is when your muscles are repaired and energy stores otherwise known as glycogen stores are replaced. Your body becomes more efficient in terms of your cardiovascular and muscular system better preparing you for your road ahead to performing more efficiently and becoming body beautiful.

Progression

Start slowly to begin with as too many people start training as if it is a race and they wonder why they cannot stick with the regime or why they get injured. You should not fall into this trap of getting carried away and ahead of yourself and instead gradually build the amount of exercise and overloading. For example increasing the resistance by even 5 kg at an appropriate time and not 15 kg to impress friends or people in the gym. As the old saying goes pride before a fall. The author has always believed that you should have enough self confidence in yourself not to worry about others and focus on the plan tailored for you. This has always brought the author great results and you will notice after weeks of dedication you are overtaking many people in the gym the proper way. Progression should be monitored regularly so as to stay on track. This is recommended every six weeks, which gives enough time for the body to adapt and the perfect time to change something if it's stopped working or make slight alterations in order to keep shocking the body into providing great results.

Reversibility

Any adaption's or gains, which have taken place as a result of exercise and your training regime will be reversed when you stop training. If you take a prolonged break or simply do not train often or consistently enough this will lead to fitness being lost. By prolonged break I mean anymore than two to three weeks for someone who is fit and has been training for quite some time. This will prove to be detrimental to their training and they will have entered into reversibility. For anyone not very fit or who is quite new to training even missing one full week could prove very detrimental to their training as they are still in the process of building their fitness levels therefore keep breaks as short as possible or if you are away on holidays or business trips for example at least do enough training to maintain your current fitness levels. Exercises, which can be carried out in your hotel room can prove very useful for maintaining fitness levels as they are not very time consuming and very convenient. I will provide some great fat burning and toning exercises later in the book, which are ideal for this.

Variation

Variety is the spice of training as well as of life in general and is the key to increasing your levels of motivation. If you do not have variety in your training regime it will not only become stale but you simply will not enjoy training, which means you will not want to commit properly to your program and therefore not achieve your goals. In order to achieve the results you want variety is one of the most important tools you will have at your disposal so use it. Variation has another important benefit in that when your body is asked to work harder or perform something different to what it normally does this takes you out of your comfort zone, which is a really good thing. This is because your body has to adapt and stretch itself in order to perform more efficiently as well as gain increased fitness and strength. Variety in your training will not only prevent staleness and hitting a wall but also will make your training a lot more enjoyable. It can also improve technical performance as some sports skills cross over very well and you can use this to refine and improve your skills in your own sport. Intensity, duration, volume, sets, reps, time and distance are all components of training which can be changed enabling you to stimulate your body into the changes you want while also making your training even more interesting. I recommend making at least a small change every six weeks and also to include variety in terms of the type of training you are doing every week.

Now that you understand what these principles mean it is up to you to apply them to your training and you will notice a considerable difference to your results. Your physique will begin to resemble the body beautiful.

CHAPTER THREE
PROGRAMS THAT WORK

Now for what you have been waiting for the author is going to give you a series of very effective programmes, which you can choose from and adapt to your own abilities while you become competent enough to perform to your maximum. The author will set out adaptable programs to cater for various types of training and exercises which can be used by many people as an effective way to get fit and lose weight.

Weight training

This is the most comprehensive resistance workout you can possibly do as it will work all your muscle groups in one total body session numerous times for greater results in super quick time. Add the finishing exercises after about six weeks when your body has adapted in terms of fitness and is better able to cope with the extra exercises. Perform this routine three times per week allowing at least 48 hours recovery between sessions. As this is a brutal workout you should listen to your body and therefore it is ok to perform the routine twice a week with lighter weights for the first two weeks as you adjust. You should aim to lift weights at around 75% of your one rep max for 6 weeks before moving up gradually. It is important to establish your one rep max in each of these exercises before you begin the program and ensure you have a training partner with you when nearing or attempting maximum lifts. These lifts will change your physique forever and take you a huge step closer to becoming body beautiful. I would say good luck but if you are disciplined enough to follow my instructions and exercises you will not need luck.

Compound moves	Sets	Repetitions
Bench press	Four sets	4-6 Strength
Bent over row		8-12 Power
Military press		12-15
Squat		Endurance
Wide grip-		
pull up		
Chin up's		
Dead lift		
Dips		
Finishing-exercises- Lunges,Lateral-raises, Shrugs,Hammer curls		
Core-Plank/Side- plank/superman-1 minute		

Circuits

These Stations are to be performed for overall fitness levels and incorporate fat loss and strength.

Lunges

Press up's

Sit up's

Military press

Squats

Bicep curls

Rows

Tricep dips

Burpees

Mountain climbers

Shuttle runs

Perform at each station for 30 seconds keeping your form throughout with 45 seconds rest between stations and 2 minutes rest after each full circuit is complete. Perform 3 full circuits in total, 2 for the first 2 weeks to give your body time to adapt. Circuits should be performed three times per week allowing at least 48 hours between sessions for recovery.

Swimming

The following session is for anyone quite new to swimming who would like to lose weight, tone up and improve their swimming. The session needs to be performed three times per week for six weeks before making alterations to ensure you keep gaining great rewards.

The following session is based on a 25 metre pool.

	Stroke	Sets-Rest.	Effort.
Warm-up		200mx1 30	3-4
Content	Breast	50mx4 30	5-6
		50mx4 20	7
		100mx1 30	6
	Freestyle	50m x1 30	8
		25m x2 10	6
	Kick-float	100m x1	2-3
		Stretch-major-	

		muscle groups.	

The following is a program designed with each workout detailed for the more advanced level swimmer who wants to progress to new levels of fitness and technique. Aim for three workouts per week in the following order.

SWIM WORKOUT 1

Warm-up. Drill Choice 300m. Freestyle

4 x 50m on 40 seconds rest 4x50m on 50

seconds rest, 4 x 50m rest for 1 minute

Kick – 200m, 8 x 25m on 40 seconds rest

Fly + Back 50m + 150m

Fly + Breast 50m + 150m

Fly + Free 50m + 150m

Choice - Pull least favourite stroke

4 x 100m

Favourite stroke 4 x 50m

Swim down - 2 x 100m

Stretch

SWIM WORKOUT 2

Warm-up - Choice 300m

Free + Choice - Kick 200m

12 x 25m 10 sec. rest, 200m,

10 x 50m rest as needed, swim 200m,

10x 75m

Drills 200m

Swim 100m

Kick 200m

Swim down - Choice 200m

Stretch

SWIM WORKOUT 3

Warm-up - Drill Choice 300m

Freestyle - 4 x 50m on: 40 seconds rest

4 x 50m on: 50, 4 x 50m On: 60

Kick 200, 8 x 25m on: 40

Fly + Back 50 + 150m

Fly + Breast 50 + 150m

Fly + Free 50 + 150m,

Choice - Pull least favourite stroke

4 x 100m

Pull favourite stroke 4 x 50m

Swim down - 2 x 100m

Stretch

SWIM WORKOUT 4

Warm-up – 500m, 1 length easy, 1 hard, 2 easy, 2 hard.

500m reverse hard to easy

Fly & Free – 100m: 25m fly, 75m free

100m: 25 free, 25mfly, 50m free

100m: 50 free, 25m fly, 25m free

100m: 75 free, 25m fly

Back & Breast - 2 x 150m: 100m back, 50m

breast 2 x 150m,

50m back, 100m breast

Free - Kick 8 x 50m on: 60

Swim 8 x 75m + 25m: moderate 75 10 sec. rest

then hard for 25m

Swim down

Free 300m

Stretch

SWIM WORKOUT 5

Warm-up - Choice non-stop Swim 100m,

Kick no board 100m, Drills 100m, Swim 100m,

25m: 25m easy fly, 75m moderate.

Free, 25m hard fly, 125m back, free, back,

125m: breast, free, breast, 125m: all free,

25m easy, 75m moderate and 25m hard.

Free + Choice - Free easy 400m

Choice hard 4 x 100m, Free easy 300m,

Choice harder 4 x 75m, Free easy 200m, Choice

hardest 4 x 50m, Free easy 100m, Choice

4 x 25m Swim down - Catch up free 200m

Stretch

SWIM WORKOUT 6

Warm-up – 500m

1 length easy, 1 hard, 2 easy, 2 hard.

500m reverse hard to easy

Fly & Free – 100m: 25m fly, 75m free 100m:

25m free, 25m fly,

50m free 100m: 50m free, 25m fly, 25m free

100m: 75m free, 25m fly

Back & Breast - 2 x 150m: 100m back,

50m breast, 2 x 150m 50m back,

100m breast

Free - Kick 8 x 50m on: 60 seconds rest

Swim 8 x 75m + 25m: Moderate 75m

10 sec. rest then hard 25m

Swim down - Pull Free 300m

Stretch

SWIM WORKOUT 7

Warm up-Drills 400 m, 1-arm Fly

Catch up free

Freestyle + Stroke - Swim Free 400m,

Swim Favourite Stroke 4x100m,

Kick Free 300m, Swim 2nd Favourite stroke

6 x 75m,

Pull Free 200m, Swim 3rd favourite stroke

8 x 50,

Swim Free 100, Swim least favourite

Stroke 8x25

Swim Down - 200

Stretch

SWIM WORKOUT 8

Warm–up-Reverse 400m free,

breast, back, fly

Free - Swim ladder 1650m 11 lengths, 10, 9,

down to 1 10 sec.

Rest between Kick 200m

Loosen up 100m

Swim 20 x 25m 5 of each stroke

Swim-down – 200m

Stretch

SWIM WORKOUT 9

Warm up Drills 400 m, 1-arm Fly

Catch up free Freestyle + Stroke –swim

Free 400m,

Swim favourite stroke 4x100m, Kick Free

300m

Swim 2nd favourite stroke 6x75

Pull Free 200m, Swim 3rd favourite stroke

8x50m,

Swim Free 100m

Swim Least Favourite Stroke 8x25m 100

Swim Down – 200m

Stretch

SWIM WORKOUT 10

Warm-Up - Swim Choice 500m

Freestyle - 2x 50m on: 45 seconds rest

2x100m on 1:30 rest,

2x 150m on 2:15 rest 1x 200 on 3:0 and 2 x

150m on 2:15

2x 100m on 1:30, 2 x 50m on: 45 seconds

rest. Backstroke - Kick & Swim 1 length kick

No board 1 length

Swim 300m

Swim 300m

Swim-down - Pull 300m

Stretch

SWIM WORKOUT 11

Warm-up

3 x 150m rest: 15 seconds rest

between 150's

Freestyle 2 x 200m: 20 seconds rest

4 x 100m: 15 seconds rest

8 x 50: 10 seconds rest

16 x 25: 5 seconds rest

Choice no free

Pull 300m

Kick 200m

Swim 15 second interval

6 x 25m no board

Swim down

SWIM WORKOUT 12

Warm-Up - Swim Choice 500

Freestyle - 2x 50m on 45 seconds rest,

2x100m on 1:30 rest

2x 150m on 2:15 rest 1x 200m on 3:0 rest

2x 150m on 2:15 rest

2x 100m on 1:30 rest 2 x 50m on 45

seconds rest

Backstroke - Kick & Swim 1 length kick no

board 1 length

Swim 300

Swim 300

Swim-down - Pull 300

Stretch

SWIM WORKOUT 13

Warm- Up - Reverse 400m

Freestyle - Swim descend 5 seconds per

swim 4x250

Backstroke - Drill 150m

Swim 200m, 8x25m on 30 seconds rest

Freestyle - Kick 300m

Pull 300m, Swim 200m

Kick no board 100m

Swim down - Free swim 150m

Stretch

SWIM WORKOUT 14

Warm-Up - Swim Choice 300m

Drills, Breast with fly kick 150m

Swim breast 100m

Kick (no board) 100m

Freestyle - 6x50m on 45 seconds rest

4x100m on 1:30 rest, 2 x100m on 3

minutes rest between

4x100m on 1:30 rest, 6 x 50m on 45

seconds rest

4x 125mRotate the 50m

Swim down - Pull choice 100m

Stretch

SWIM WORKOUT 15

Warm- Up - Reverse 400

Freestyle - Swim descend 5 seconds per

swim 4x250m

Backstroke - Drill 150m,

Swim 200m

8x25m on 30 seconds rest

Freestyle - Kick 300m

Pull 300m, Swim 200m

Kick no board 100m

Swim down - Free swim 150m

Stretch

SWIM WORKOUT 16

Warm-up - Free Drills - one arm, catch-up,

ripple, and choice 400m

Freestyle + 200m

1st 25m fly, rest free 200m

2nd 25m backstroke, rest free 200m

3rd 25m breaststroke, rest free 200m

Choice - the entire same stroke 10 x 75m,

1st 5, rest 10 seconds 2nd 5, rest 15

Seconds Free - Pull 1 length normal

breathing, 1 length minimal breathing

500m, Swim all out 2x50m

Swim-down 250m

Stretch

SWIM WORKOUT 17

Warm-up - Swim choice 300m

Free - Swim time trial, 5 seconds slower

100m 5 x 100m on 1:30 rest 5 x 100m on

1:45 rest. Butterfly - Drills 1 arm, kick with

arms in stream line 200m

4 x 25m on: 60 seconds rest, 4 x 25m on 45

seconds rest

Backstroke-Drills 1 stroke, kick on side,

other arm kick

200m, 8x25m on 35 seconds rest

Breaststroke - Drills 1 stroke, 2kicks, 2

strokes, 1 kick,

fly kick 200

8x25m on 40 seconds rest

Freestyle - Drills 1 arm, catch-up 200

8x 25m on

30 seconds rest

Swim-down - Pull choice 200m

Stretch

SWIM WORKOUT 18

Warm-up - Free Drills- one arm, catch-up,

ripple, choice 400m

Freestyle + 200m 1st 25m fly, rest free

200m, 2nd 25m backstroke, rest free 200m,

3rd 25m breaststroke, rest free 200m

Choice - All the same stroke 10 x 75, 1st 5,

rest 10 seconds

2nd 5m, rest 15 seconds

Free -Pull 1 length normal breathing,

1 length minimal breathing

500m

Swim all out - 2x50m

Swim-down – 250m

Stretch

Running programs for 5k and 10 k

5 km for beginners

Run at a pace where you can hold conversation.

Week 1

Monday-rest day.

Tuesday-Run 1 minute, walk 2 minutes repeat x 6.

Wednesday-rest day.

Thursday- Run 1 minute, walk 2 minutes and repeat x 6.

Friday-Rest day.

Saturday- Rest day.

Sunday- Run 1 minute, walk 1 minute and repeat x 6.

Week 2

Monday-Rest day.

Tuesday-Run 2 minutes, walk 4 minutes and repeat x 5.

Wednesday-Rest day.

Thursday-Run 1 minute, walk 1 minute and repeat x 10.

Friday-Rest day.

Saturday-Rest day.

Sunday- Run 1 mile and record your time.

Week 3

Monday-Rest day.

Tuesday- Run 3 minutes, walk 3 minutes and repeat x 4.

Wednesday-Rest day.

Thursday- Run 3 minutes, walk 3 minutes and repeat x 4.

Friday-Rest day.

Saturday-Rest day.

Sunday- Run 3 minutes, walk 2 minutes and repeat x 5.

Week 4

Monday-Rest day.

Tuesday-Run 5 minute's walk 3 minutes and repeat this x 3.

Wednesday-Rest day.

Thursday-Run 5 minute's walk 3 minutes and repeat x 3.

Friday-Rest day.

Saturday-Rest day.

Sunday- Run and walk 1 mile and repeat.

Again record your time.

Week 5

Monday-Rest day.

Tuesday- Run 7 minutes, walk 2 minutes and repeat x 3.

Wednesday-Rest day.

Thursday- Run 7 minutes, walk 2 minutes and repeat x 3.

Friday-Rest day.

Saturday-Rest day.

Sunday-Run 8 minutes, walk 2 minutes and repeat x 3.

Week 6

Monday-Rest day.

Tuesday-Run 8 minutes, walk 2 minutes and repeat x 3.

Wednesday-Rest day.

Thursday- Run 10 minutes, walk 2minutes and repeat x 2.

Friday-Rest day.

Saturday-Rest day.

Sunday- Run 1 mile, walk 1 mile.

Record your time.

Week 7

Monday-Rest day.

Tuesday-Run 12 minutes walk 2 minutes x 2.

Wednesday-Rest day.

Thursday- Run 12 minutes, walk 2 minutes, repeat x 2.

Friday-Rest day.

Saturday-Rest day.

Sunday- Run 2 miles and record your time.

Week 8

Monday-Rest day.

Tuesday-Run 15 minute's walk 2 and repeat x 2.

Wednesday-Rest day.

Thursday-Run 15 minute's walk 2 and repeat x 2.

Friday-Rest day.

Saturday-Rest day.

Sunday- Run 2 mile, walk and jog 1 mile.

Record your time. You are now ready to run a 5 km race.

10km training program.

You should be able to hold a conversation while performing the runs in this program.

Week 1

Monday- Rest day.

Tuesday- 1.5 mile run.

Wednesday- Bike for 40 minutes easy pace or rest depending on how you feel.

Thursday- 1.5 mile run.

Friday- Rest day.

Saturday- 2 mile run.

Sunday- 25 minute's walk and run.

Week 2

Monday- Rest day.

Tuesday- 2 mile run.

Wednesday- Bike 40 minutes easy to moderate pace or rest completely.

Thursday- 2 mile run.

Friday- Rest day.

Saturday- 2.5 mile run.

Sunday- 30 minutes cross trainer.

Week 3

Monday- Rest day.

Tuesday- 2.5 mile run.

Wednesday- Bike 45 minutes easy pace.

Thursday- 2 mile run.

Friday- Rest day.

Saturday- 3.5 mile run.

Sunday-Cross-trainer 1.5 miles easy pace.

Week 4

Monday- Rest day.

Tuesday- 2.5 mile run.

Wednesday- Bike 45 minutes easy to

moderate pace.

Thursday- 2 mile run.

Friday- Rest day.

Saturday- 3.5 mile run.

Sunday- 35 minute's walk and run

alternating each for 5 minutes.

Week 5

Monday- Rest day.

Tuesday- 3 mile run.

Wednesday- Bike 35 minutes moderate pace.

Thursday- 2 mile run.

Friday- Rest day.

Saturday- 4 mile run.

Sunday- 40 minute's walk and run alternating each for 5 minutes.

Week 6

Monday- Rest day.

Tuesday- 3 mile run.

Wednesday- Bike 45 minutes moderate pace.

Thursday- 2.5 mile run.

Friday- Rest day.

Saturday- 4.5 mile run.

Sunday- 35 minute's walk.

Week 7

Monday- Rest day.

Tuesday- 3.5 mile run.

Wednesday- Bike 50 minutes easy pace.

Thursday- 3 mile run.

Friday- Rest day.

Saturday 5 mile run.

Sunday- Walk and run for 40 minutes

alternating each every 5 minutes.

Week 8

Monday- Rest day.

Tuesday- 3 mile run.

Wednesday- Bike 45 minutes easy pace.

Thursday- 2 mile run.

Friday- Rest day.

Saturday- Rest day.

Sunday- You are ready for your first 10km race.

Exercise programs for a Tennis club player and a professional player

Professional Tennis player- Cardio

Perform the following routine twice per week allowing at least 48 hours for recovery. This obviously is in addition to your tennis practice.

Warm up- Run 1 mile at an easy pace followed by alternating lunges as you are moving around 12 on each leg x 3. 400m x 3 at an easy pace with a 1 minute break between.

Content. The author is choosing 400m runs to base this session on as it improves lactic acid removal dramatically. 400m x 8 giving yourself 80 seconds maximum to complete each 400m and 2 minutes to recover in between.

Cool down- Run 1 mile slowly.

Professional-Player Strength

Warm up by performing all the lifts 10 repetitions each without any weight on the bar.

Perform the following exercises 3 times per week for 6 sets of 5 repetitions.

Back squat

Box jumps

Walking lunges.

Cycle split jump

Pull ups

5kg medicine ball throw-down

Dips

5kg medicine ball chest pass

Lateral side lunges

Max distance lateral hops

Cable woodchop

5 kg medicine ball throws

Power clean

Tennis club player program

Cardio

Choose whichever day's that suit you as long as there is a 48 hour recovery period in between and your session is endurance based choosing from cycling, swimming and running. The author's advice would be to cycle despite swimming being a great form of exercise as the upper body muscles will be worked enough with the resistance program involved here and running can be very sore on the joints when it is added to the running and drills already involved in your tennis sessions. Cycling will not only prepare your leg muscles for the competition ahead but also build superior strength, power and definition without unnecessary pressure on your joints.

You should aim for 45 minutes at a moderate pace, which will work but you should still be able to hold a conversation. This should be your aim for the first 4 weeks and then increase the duration of exercise to 55 minutes from week's 4-8 at a pace slightly higher than moderate. This is between 90-100 rpm for most people.

Throughout this period you should aim to play tennis for no more than an hour three times a week concentrating only on specific drills aimed at improving areas of weakness and maintaining areas of strength. You should start to include practice sets and increase the frequency of tennis practice after the initial eight weeks training.

You should have one day per week to rest completely to allow your body time to recover.

Resistance-Tennis club player

Monday, Wednesday and Fridays will be the days that you will work on your resistance exercises. You should try to ensure that your session's lasts no longer than 50 minutes each day as this will be detrimental to your performance and results. You should include the following lifts and exercises;

Warm up by replicating the movements below using only the barbells without weight or very light dumbbells for 10 repetitions for each.

Main session. Perform in the following order for the first 4 weeks then change the order and weight for weeks 4-8. Aim to perform the following exercises for 3 sets of 8 repetitions.

Back extensions

Bench press

Single armed rows

Squats

Military presses

Lunges

Pull ups wide grip

Calf raises

Press ups

Upright rows

Shoulder extensions- lateral raises

Forearm pronation and supination

Wrist curls and extensions

Bicep curls

Core- Criss cross sit ups. Plank 1 minute x 3.

Once you begin playing competitively you should reduce resistance training to twice per week and stop all forms of training during tournament weeks so as maintain enough energy reserves.

Programs-Cycling club amateur and professional cyclist.

Club Cyclist

You must find out what your MHR is.

Week 1

Sunday-Road. Warm up for 10 minutes at low intensity and steady pace between 85-110 revolutions per minute (RPM). Continue to ride at this pace using a gear ratio of 42-15 for 2 hours on flat roads.

Monday-Rest day.

Tuesday-Road. Warm up for 7 minutes then ride at a pace between 90-100 rpms about 70-75% of maximum heart rate (MHR) using a 42-15 gear ratio for 1 ½ hours again on flat roads.

Wednesday-Turbo. Warm up for 7 minutes then ride using a gear ratio of 42-15 at a steady pace of between 90-100 rpms, this is around 70-75% of maximum heart rate for 45 minutes.

Thursday-Turbo. Set resistance to very low on your trainer. Warm up slowly for 7 minutes. Then increase your gear to around 42x16 and pedal at around 110 rpm for 50 seconds. Ride easy for 2 minutes to recover. Repeat this for 50 minutes have passed. Warm down for 5 minutes.

Friday-Turbo. Warm up for 12 minutes at an easy pace using a gear ratio of 42-17. Keep riding at this pace about 85-90 rpm for 45 minutes.

Saturday-Rest day.

Week 2

Sunday-Road. Warm up for 12 minutes gradually. Ride using the gear ratio 42-15 for 2 hours 10 minutes at this intensity between 85-105 rpm 75-80% of maximum heart rate level on flat roads.

Monday-Rest day.

Tuesday-Road. Warm up for 7 minutes gradually. Ride for 1 hour 45 minutes at an intensity of between 90-100 rpm about 75% of maximum heart rate using 42-15 gear ratio.

Wednesday-Turbo. Warm-up-7 minutes. Ride for 45 minutes using gear 42-15 between 90-100 rpm. Cool down for 5 minutes.

Thursday-Turbo. Set resistance to very low on your trainer and use gear ratio 42-17. Warm up for 7 minutes then increase you cadence slightly to between 105-115 rpm for 50 seconds. Ride easy for 2 minutes to recover. Repeat until 30 minutes have passed. Cool down for 5 minutes.

Friday-Turbo. Warm up for 12 minutes. Then ride using gear ratio of 42-15 for 45 minutes at an intensity of between 90-100 rpm. Cool down for 5 minutes to complete the session.

Saturday-Rest day.

Week 3

Sunday-Road. Warm up for 12 minutes. Ride at a low level intensity using 42-15 gear ratio at a pace between 85-100 rpm about 75% of maximum effort for 2 hours 30 minutes on flat roads.

Monday-Rest day.

Tuesday-Road. Warm up for 7 minutes. Ride using 42-15 gear for 1 hour 30 minutes again on flat roads at an intensity of between 90-100 rpm about 75% MHR. Cool down for 5 minutes.

Wednesday-Turbo. Warm up for 5 minutes gradually then ride using 42-15 gear for 40 minutes at an intensity of between 90-100 rpm.

Thursday-Turbo. Set resistance to very low on your trainer and use 42-17 gear ratio. Warm up for 7 minutes. Ride at an intensity of between 105-115, which is about 85% of MHR for 45 seconds then ride very easy for 2 minutes to recover. Repeat until 50 minutes have elapsed. Cool down for 5 minutes.

Friday-Turbo. Warm up for 12 minutes then ride in 42-15 gear for 45 minutes at a steady pace between 90-100 rpm about 75% of maximum heart rate. 5 minute cool down.

Saturday-Rest day.

Week 4

Sunday-Road. Warm up for 12 minutes and then ride in 42-15 gear for 2 hours 25 minutes on flat roads at an intensity between 85-105 rpm about 75-80% of maximum heart rate.

Monday-Rest day.

Tuesday-Road. Warm up for 7 minutes then ride in 42-15 gear for 2 hours at between 90-100 rpm. Cool down for 5 minutes.

Wednesday-Turbo. Warm up for 7 minutes gradually. Ride for 1 hour in 42-15 gear at an intensity between 90-100 rpm about 75% of your maximum heart rate. Cool down for 6 minutes.

Thursday-Turbo. Set resistance to very low on the trainer and your gear to 42-15. Warm up for 7 minutes gradually. Increase cadence to between 105-120 rpm about 85% of maximum heart rate for 45 seconds then cycle easy for 2 minutes. Repeat until 30 minutes have elapsed. Cool down for 6 minutes.

Friday-Turbo. Warm up for 12 minutes gradually. Ride in 42-15 gear for 1 hour at an intensity between 90-100 rpm about 75% of MHR. Cool down for 6 minutes.

Saturday-Rest day.

Week 5

Sunday-Road. Warm up for 12 minutes. Ride for 2 hours 50 minutes the first half between 85-100 rpm about 75% and the second half of your journey at 80% of you maximum heart rate on flat roads.

Monday Rest day.

Tuesday-Road. Warm up for 7 minutes then cycle in 42-15 gear for 2 hours 15 minutes at between 90-100 rpm. Cool down for 5 minutes.

Wednesday-Turbo. Set resistance very low again and use 42-17 gear. Warm up for 7 minutes the increase cadence to 115 rpm for 40 seconds, which should be around 85-90% of your maximum. Ride easy for 2 minutes and repeat until 30 minutes have elapsed. Cool down for 3 minutes.

Thursday-Turbo. Warm up for 7 minutes the cycle in 42-15 gear for 1 hour between 90-100 rpm. Cool down for 6 minutes.

Friday-Turbo. Warm up for 12 minutes. Ride in 53-17 gear for 30 minutes at an intensity of 80-90 rpm about 65-70% and the ride in 42-15 gear for another 30 minutes at an intensity of 90-100 rpm about 75% of MHR. Cool down for 5 minutes.

Saturday-Rest day.

Week 6

Sunday-Road. Warm up for 12 minutes. Cycle in 42-15 gear for 3 hours 15 minutes on flat roads at intensity between 85-100 rpm, which is around 75%.

Monday-Rest day.

Tuesday-Road. Warm up for 7 minutes. Ride for 2 hours 20 minutes again on flat roads at an intensity between 90-100 rpm 75% of MHR for the first 1 hour 35 minutes then at an intensity of 80% for the remaining 45 minutes.

Wednesday-Turbo. Set Resistance at very low on your trainer and use gear 42-17. Warm up for 7 minutes. Increase cadence to 115 rpm for 45 seconds then cycle easy for 2 minutes. Repeat until 30 minutes have elapsed. Cool down for 5 minutes.

Thursday-Turbo. Warm up for 7 minutes. Ride in 42-15 gear for 1 hour between 90-100 rpm. Cool down for 5 minutes.

Friday-Turbo. Warm up for 12 minutes. Ride in 53-17 gear for 45 minutes between 65-70 rpm and then for 15 minutes at 75-80% of maximum heart rate.

Saturday-Rest day.

Professional cyclist

Top fitness components for cycling include stamina, strength, skill, aerobic and anaerobic power, specificity and speed. Specificity to the demands or goals of cycling must be fundamental or you are limiting your potential. You must maintain and improve areas you are already strong in but even more importantly improve your weaker areas otherwise you or your times will not reach your full potential. The following are training sessions good enough to be used by top professionals and you can tailor any of them to your needs.

First workout

Perform a 1 hour 50 minute ride that has some five-minute intervals about 85-90% of your maximum effort for the last 3 minutes. Try to maintain this pace. You should perform five intervals of five minutes and each one beginning with a 25 second sprint. Ride easy for the next one minute 35 seconds and then perform three minutes at 85-90% of your maximum.

Second workout

Another good session to use is an interval session where you perform for 20 seconds on, 40 seconds off. Do these on a slight incline so even in the 40 seconds off you still have to work hard? Perform 4 sets of these. Try to find a hill which is not to steep and takes around 8 minutes to climb. After a 20 minute warm up begin cycling up the hill for 2 minutes then begin your intervals until you reach the top and free wheel back down after a short rest. Repeat this 3 times for first few sessions then progress it to 4.

Third workout

A 3 hour 45 minute ride with two huge efforts during a long climb in a mountainous area. Monitor your average watts and time on the climb to see how you are going. Do not ride at your threshold all the way and the two huge efforts should not last longer than 15 minutes each with a gap of 1 hour between. What you should do is ride just below your threshold then raise your effort levels to slightly above and back off to just below your threshold throughout both the 15 minute periods each time you perform this session. The session tells you how you are going because you will have power outputs and times to compare. These efforts when already riding at a high level create a lot of lactate in the muscles, because of the anaerobic nature of the training. But when you drop back under your threshold the body has to clear the lactate and recover while still maintaining a high pace, which is ideal for race preparation. Once per week is enough for this particular session at least until you join the professional ranks.

Forth workout

You will need a power meter or a turbo with power readout for the following session. Warm up for about 12 minutes and set one is also 12 minutes this time performing 10 seconds at 150 to 200 watts above 10 mile time trial power alternated with 20 seconds riding very easy or complete rest. Set two is eight minutes of 15 seconds between 90 to 100 watts above 10-mile time trial power alternated with 15 seconds very easy or rest. Set three is four minutes of 40 seconds at around 70 to 80 watts above 10 mile time trial power alternated with 20 seconds very easy or complete rest. Follow this with 8 minutes easy pedalling to cool-down effectively.

Fifth workout

This workout is short and not so sweet but it works. After a 5 minute warm up you ride for 25 minutes just under your anaerobic threshold. Then go into intervals, where you ride as fast as you can for one minute and then recover for two minutes. Perform 8- 10 of these intervals starting with 4-5 for the first few sessions.

Fat burners.

Perform the following exercises four times per week. Choose from the exercises below beginning with star jumps and do not choose more than four to begin with. Perform each one for 30 seconds continuously until all four exercises are complete then rest for one minute. Repeat this three times in each session for the first four weeks then increase to four times per session for weeks four to eight. Change your choice and order of exercises every four weeks in order to shock your body into producing great results on a consistent basis. For those of you with limited time to train these are a very smart and efficient way to get into and stay in shape as you are only working out for six and eight minutes per day four times per week. Now know one can use time as an excuse preventing you from being in great shape and off course being body beautiful.

Mountain climbers

Burpees

Spiderman press ups

Skipping

Sprinting on the spot using high knees

Star jumps

Alternating knee to elbow power drives

Squats

Squats to military press

Kettle bell swings

Lateral hops

Walking Lunges

Tricep dips

Stretching exercises

Static and dynamic

Core exercises-Criss cross, plank and

side plank, Swiss ball sit up and cradle boat.

CHAPTER FOUR
COMPONENTS OF FITNESS

Now for something very important to think about when designing a program, which many people and trainers do not always take into account. This can be for various reasons such as some people tend to obsess over one goal where they will focus on becoming stronger ignoring all the other areas where they could use improvement or some trainers may not have the knowledge or experience to balance the program they are designing while still meeting the clients goals. This very important aspect of fitness training and program design that I am referring to is known simply as the components of fitness. When many people talk about their own or others levels of fitness you will often hear people say things like he is really thin, he has very big muscles, he or she is so toned, he runs four or five times a week, I just want to get stronger and bigger, I just want to lose weight or he can run really far. These types of statements show very limited understanding of fitness training as just because someone excels at one thing does not mean they would perform very well at all if asked to perform another task or exercise. Many people if asked to perform a variety of fitness tests would be quite surprised to see just how much they need to improve certain aspects of their fitness. Fitness is an ability to perform a task efficiently and effectively meeting the demands of your sport or training regime. Fitness is also used to improve you holistically in terms of your confidence, physically and mentally, quality of life, health, skills, socially as well as to incorporate as many of the components as possible.

The components of fitness are as follows;

-aerobic and anaerobic fitness

-muscular endurance

-flexibility

-strength

-agility

-speed

-power

Aerobic endurance (Stamina)

Aerobic endurance refers to the ability of the cardiovascular otherwise known as the respiratory systems to supply the muscles being utilised in exercise with the oxygen needed to sustain aerobic exercise for quite long periods of time, for example swimming for an hour or running a marathon. Possessing good levels of aerobic endurance can help when carrying out daily activities as you're not as tired but are very important for participating or competing in sports such as cycling, swimming and running. Anaerobic fitness refers to training and sports which involve periods of oxygen debt. For example when sprinting a 100m the athlete is effectively not breathing properly because they simply cannot take in enough oxygen to supply the muscles under stress over short periods of time therefore creating lactic acid in the body. Anaerobic training is necessary for any sport where there is sprinting or interval work involved.

Muscular endurance

Muscular endurance is the ability to perform repeated muscle contractions for sustained periods of time. For example swimming and press ups. This is obviously a very important component of fitness as without development an athlete would be unable to perform repeated movements, techniques and actions their sport demands on a consistent basis meaning levels would drop to well below that of a professional. This is a vital element which must not be overlooked by athletes or the amateur trainer.

Flexibility

Flexibility is the ability your joints have to move through a full range of movement and is very important for both the sports you play and your health. I have seen many people completely ignore their own flexibility when training leaving no time in their workouts to improve it. There are two types of flexibility: Static and Dynamic. Dynamic flexibility is the range of movement a muscle or joint can perform while moving and can be limited by current levels of static flexibility and co-ordination. Static flexibility is the range of movement a muscle or joint can perform from stationary positions and can be limited by the structure of your joints, bones as well as muscle tone and size. Poor flexibility usually results in injury, which is why it is important to ensure you leave some time in your workouts for stretching.

Strength

Strength is a single maximal contraction of force by specific muscles. This is used in weight lifting as well as in many other sports to varying degrees. The force created is used to overcome a chosen form of resistance. Strength is another component, which is often overlooked as people tend to associate strength with weight lifters and body builders not realising it is an essential component in most sports and should be developed by any athlete or trainer serious about their own personal goals. It is possible to build serious strength without looking too big.

Agility

Agility is the ability to change direction, twist and turn quickly enabling you to get into position better. This is very evident in top tennis players where they constantly have to change direction in order to stay in and win rallies. In order to improve agility it requires many drills as well as natural attributes such as speed, co-ordination and flexibility.

Speed

Speed is an ability to move over distances in a short space of time. Speed is needed by many athletes and sports stars to improve their performance and can give them a real advantage. For example a footballer who can beat another player in a race to the ball can create a scoring opportunity. The 100m and other forms of sprinting is an obvious example where an athlete will try to maximise their speed in order to get an advantage over their competitors. Speed endurance, which is a combination of speed and endurance is another form of speed whereby an athlete is expected to make a series of repeated sprints and this would be necessary in the training of both the afore mentioned examples.

Power

Power is when an athlete can produce and effectively use muscle strength with speed in a short amount of time. Power is a very necessary element for many sports and requires more advanced training methods. For example Resistance band work for practising a golf swing or tennis serve and bag work in order to deliver an effective punch in boxing.

Should all these elements be included in your workouts you will not only look and feel great but also have a superb balance of fitness, which others will find difficult to match. This in turn will aid your performance in a variety of activities and sports increasing your confidence to whole new levels.

CHAPTER FIVE
NUTRITION

A healthy balanced diet is crucial for any athlete in order to improve performance and is an essential element in an athlete's lifestyle and overall health and well being. Just as a car needs fuel in order to function and perform an athlete needs the best fuel to function effectively and perform at optimum levels. Carbohydrates are an important energy source and can be accessed quickly when required. There are a couple of types of carbohydrate. These include simple carbohydrates made up of sugary foods such as jams, honey, minerals, sweets, energy gels and fruit juices, which are easily digested, absorbed and provide energy fast. Glucose will also give you energy fast and can be used to produce adenosine triphosphate also known as ATP, which is basically an energy currency. This currency is essential for training at optimum levels. The other type of carbohydrates is complex carbohydrates, which are digested and released slowly over extended periods. These types of Carbohydrates should make up the majority of peoples carbohydrate intake. You should stick to the unrefined versions which include wholegrain pastas, oats, rice, noodles, and cereal and whole meal type breads. Glycogen stores in your muscles and liver are extracted from eating carbohydrates and these can be easily used when you need energy therefore it is important that you eat carbohydrates ensuring you choose the correct types. A great tip to remember is by eating some carbohydrates post exercise within an hour of training is beneficial to recovery and replacing glycogen stores. About 60-70% of your daily intake should be carbohydrates. Carbohydrate intake breaks down as follows; 1 gram of carbohydrate = 4 kcal of energy.

An aerobic athlete should aim to maximise glycogen stores by eating carbohydrates especially in the run up to an event. For example from about three days before competition an athlete should increase carbohydrate consumption.

Anaerobic athletes should combine carbohydrate intake which is still important with protein within an hour post exercise in order to increase protein synthesis and thus aid muscle rebuilding and development. Carbohydrate intake is also important for strength and endurance sports.

Proteins especially those containing all twenty amino acids are vital in order for muscles to function correctly repair and grow. Out of the twenty amino acids there are eight which need to come from your diet as your body can make up the rest. Protein can be used as a secondary energy source if your body is lacking carbohydrates and fats. Protein should be taken on a daily basis as it cannot be stored like carbohydrates however too much protein can be converted into fat. A typical portion of protein should be about the size of your fist to ensure your body is receiving adequate amounts. Foods which contain the eight essential amino acids are meat, eggs, fish, milk, cheese, soya, poultry and offal. In order to recover properly from any training session it is essential that you do not neglect your protein intake and you will reap the rewards and will be on your way to being body beautiful. About 15-20% of your daily intake should be protein.

Fats in moderation are essential to us all every day, which may come as a surprise to some of you as they not only provide very concentrated sources of energy but also protect our vital organs. Fats can be separated into saturated and unsaturated. Saturated fats would be found in foods such as butter, meat, eggs and dairy. Unsaturated fats are found in liquids like sunflower and olive oils. You can especially if you are an athlete cut back a little on your fats and eat extra carbohydrates which will aid both training and competition. Aim for around 25-30% 6% saturated fats of your daily food intake to be fats.

Vitamins are crucial in the correct amount. A good balanced diet and a good multi vitamin will ensure your body will not suffer from any deficiencies. Vitamins should be taken on a daily basis as they perform a variety of functions such as metabolic processes including energy release, immune, nervous system support as well as helping with muscle growth. Age, sex, level of activity and health play a part in which vitamins you require, however a balanced and varied diet should provide most of what you need. Consult with a good pharmacist when choosing a multi vitamin and these will provide you with any vitamins and minerals you are not receiving.

Minerals are also important for your health and are required daily by your body. There are two types of minerals Macro minerals such as calcium and trace elements such as selenium. Minerals are also needed for bone, connective tissue, enzymes and hormones. Minerals also help to balance fluids and with muscle contractions. Your body absorbs and excretes them so as you have just the correct balance of minerals.

Fibre is a type of food which cannot be digested and helps transport food through your digestive system for excretion. Whole grains, nuts, fruit and vegetables are all good fibre providers. Eating fibre can prevent certain cancers and keep your bowel functioning to its optimum capacity. Off course this is aided by drinking plenty of water which is as essential in its own rite as eating any of the foods mentioned. Monitoring your food intake is important as your requirements may change depending on the time of year it is with regard to training and competition. Pre season needs depend on the intensity of the training but do tend to prioritise the shedding of post season weight gain. Mid season requirements would ensure you are getting enough energy and fluid from your diet and would have specific requirements for pre -post competition in order to maximise performance and recovery. Post season is a time when the athlete can relax their usually strict regime a little but will have to be careful not to put on much weight. A good pre competition meal would usually consist of carbohydrates, some protein, very low amounts of fat and protein and should be food that you already eat regularly and have no digestive problems with. This should be taken with about two and a half hours to go before your event. It is also very important to consume plenty of fluids before, during and after exercise or competition. As soon as you complete your event carbohydrates should then be consumed within half an hour if possible as this is when the muscles capacity to refuel and start rebuilding is at its greatest level. Obviously it is not always practical to get the chance to eat so quickly however you should try to at least have a carbohydrate snack with you. Your next meal usually your dinner or a larger meal should also be carbohydrate rich and be consumed within two hours to aid recovery. Many people discuss their weight but surprisingly many fail to distinguish between actual gains in fat or muscle as both are illustrated on the scales. Muscle gain will show as weight but it will obviously not have the repercussions that gains in fat will have. Therefore it is more important to look at your body fat percentage rather than become obsessed by your body weight. Overall the author's advice would be to stick to fresh foods such as fruits, vegetables, nuts, meats and fish avoiding packaged or processed foods. Off course you can have a couple of treats per week if you are eating healthy the rest of the time and this will avoid bad cravings and binge eating. By eating fresh foods you will have the carbohydrates, proteins and fats you need without the weight gain and sometimes harmful ingredients other foods give you. You should also try to eat breakfast every morning as this boosts your metabolism, eat regularly throughout the day every two to three hours including snacks and drink plenty of water. Avoid alcohol as this is empty calories and a harmful drug if not taken in moderation, smoking of any kind and also try not to eat late in the evenings. Should you follow these guidelines you will feel great and will be a huge step closer to becoming part of the body beautiful?

CHAPTER SIX
LIFESTYLE

In order to become a successful athlete or even attain the body of an athlete sacrifices must be made. This usually comes down to lifestyle. Activities conducive to an athlete and your lifestyle for best results are resting to allow your body and mind time to recover properly. Obviously many people will have working and family commitments but by allowing time for relaxation and a proper night's sleep every day then you will be ahead of the pack. Activities such as going to the cinema, theatre, restaurant, yoga or watching television in moderation are ideal forms of relaxation. Activities, which are not a good choice for any lifestyle never mind an athletes are smoking, drinking alcohol and gambling. Binge drinking in particular can create many problems such as contributing to liver damage, heart disease, cancer, weight gain, anti-social behaviour and inability to perform to your very best in sports. Performance enhancing or recreational drugs can have severe side effects and should be avoided. Gambling can also be a major problem especially for people and athletes with plenty of money and time on their hands. This is another vice, which needs to be avoided as it has untold problems such as financial hardship through loosing large sums of money, stress, addiction, family problems, lack of focus and control of your life. You should off course ensure you spend time with family and good friends but think twice before continuing to hang out with anyone involved with gambling, or has consistently bad habits and behaviour, excessive drinkers and drug takers as this influence will only drag you and your performance down. Hang with like-minded supportive people. Think about your own motivation levels and what really makes you tick and drives you forward. Be honest with yourself and then you can use this information to ensure you stay motivated in the future. Stress can impact your performance as if you allow yourself to get worked up or want something too much this can cause something known as over arousal, which has a detrimental effect on performance. Set yourself goals short, medium and long term, which are realistic and you can achieve if you put your mind to it. Do not be afraid of making mistakes as we all do, just keep going unless you are injured. Plan, organise and manage your lifestyle to keep control. Of course you will still have to adapt but this is a less stressful method to live by. Communicate effectively with others and do not bottle everything up regarding sport, training or personal life. Talk to someone you can trust be that a professional or peers who understand where you are coming from who share similar goals and aspirations. Try to have a career plan if you want to take sport, training to professional level. You can use a Swot analysis to help with this, which is simply listing your strengths, weaknesses, opportunities and possible threats to your training and sporting aspirations. Now you can use this book and the tools it has given you to build your confidence get fit and live the life you want and deserve. Remember to post a nice review for my book. Should you have any questions or simply want to get in touch you can contact the author by sending any of your queries and comments via e-mail to barryludlowbodybeautiful1@gmail.com